Homemade Medical Face Mask

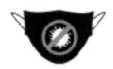

How to Make Your Own DIY Face Mask at Home. A Quick Guide for Sanitize and Protect Yourself and Your Family from Viruses and Infections.

Tom Jones

writing from the publisher except in the case of brief quotations embodied in critical articles or reviews.

Legal & Disclaimer

The information contained in this book and its contents is not designed to replace or take the place of any form of medical or professional advice; and is not meant to replace the need for independent medical, financial, legal or other professional advice or services, as may be required. The content and information in this book has been provided for educational and entertainment purposes only.

The content and information contained in this book has been compiled from sources deemed reliable, and it is accurate to the best of the Author's knowledge, information and belief. However, the Author cannot guarantee its accuracy and validity and cannot be held liable for any errors and/or omissions. Further, changes are periodically made to this book as and when needed. Where appropriate and/or necessary, you must consult a professional (including but not limited to your doctor, attorney, financial advisor or such other professional advisor) before using any of the suggested remedies, techniques, or information in this book.

Upon using the contents and information contained in this book, you agree to hold harmless the Author from and against any damages, costs, and expenses, including any legal fees potentially resulting from the application of any of the information provided by this book. This disclaimer applies to any loss, damages or injury caused by the use and application, whether directly or indirectly, of any advice or information presented, whether for breach of contract, tort, negligence, personal injury, criminal intent, or under any other cause of action.

You agree to accept all risks of using the information presented inside this book.

You agree that by continuing to read this book, where appropriate and/or necessary, you shall consult a professional (including but not limited to your doctor, attorney, or financial advisor or such other advisor as needed) before using any of the suggested remedies, techniques, or information in this book.

TABLE OF CONTENT

INTRODUCTION

In times like this, protecting our heath has to be at the center of our concern. Though many of us, have already been placed in some form of quarantine scenario, the reality is there will still be instances that you may be forced to go out into the public. This could be a simple trip to the grocery store, hospital or even an unfortunate scenario such as a fire alarm that requires you to exit the safe space you have created.

In these cases, the need for a protective mask multiplies. Luckily, there are a bunch of simple techniques that can be utilized to create protective masks using everyday home supplies that should be easy to attain. I have included the best methods that I have found below, and have also done my best to pass on whatever knowledge I have learned to employ for myself, to hopeful help you keep yourself, children and other family members safe. Let's jump right in, shall we?

Face masks are a sort of sanitary protection. There are numerous types of masks that can be categorized according to design, use, form, and mask safety.

Where the interchangeable face did masks come from then? What is the role of disposable facial masks?

In 1895 a German pathologist study showed that an infectious infection was related to a patient's injury. He claimed the sputum would contain bacteria and induce wound contamination while people were talking. Despite his advice, doctors and nurses put on the gauze edge at that time. A nose- and mouth mask can prevent wound infection during surgery. Since then, the medical personnel, food hygiene and sales personnel, and the canteen cooks have been used frequently with disposable facial masks, especially as food production and sales personnel work.

Surgical personnel shall wear a protective mask to shield patients from surgical accident infections. Medical-surgical masks are designed to protect medical or allied staff from leaking blood, body fluids, and spread during invasive procedures. Environmental health workers and employers in dusty offices also have to wear dust masks, which are also openly identified with job benefits. In the general public, especially in the flu season, there are many people wearing anti-fog masks who have, in fact, played a positive role in preventing disease spread.

From the physiological point of view, a lot of pollen, bacteria, viruses, and various toxic substances are found in the air, which can penetrate the nose, pharynx, and trachea with human breath. If people are weak, it can cause disease. The use of a disposable mask is like the 'barrier' to the respiratory tract, to allow the inhaled air to clean out and to avoid the entrance of viruses and bacteria into the body. At the same time, a mask can also protect the mouth and nose from bacteria and viruses. It is also a common norm to kill others when you cough or sneeze.

Wearing a disposable face mask may also decrease or avoid the stimulation of dust of the respiratory tract that can deter or reduce the incidence of occupational diseases. Anti-virus masks should be used in the workplace with dangerous and hazardous chemical scents to avoid industrial diseases caused by inhalation of poisonous and harmful chemicals, such as benzene poisoning and organic solvent toxicity.

Face Masks in China normally, it isn't a good sign that the most difficult product of the season is a face mask. With China battling the spread of a new Cvirus killed 1,114 people and had sickened 44,000 by Feb. 12, Face Mask factories across the world have been operating for weeks to hold demand up. However, materials tend to be low enough for local governments to requisition imports for other cities, and people in certain areas have to apply for government coupons if they want to take any hands.

Between pervasive air pollution and sporadic disease outbreak, photos of Chinese people face blurred in the last 40 years of breakneck growth have become a kind of visual deficiency for certain issues. However, it is an ongoing project for all its obvious ubiquity to convince the public to really wear the masks. In the early days of the current outbreak, networks left an episode of commentaries moaning that their parents and aged relatives are having difficulties masking as they leave. The masks you see on the streets of China are the products of a deliberate centuries-long campaign to boost national grooming and health standards.

Long before anything like a face mask was created, China simply covered her mouth with her sleeves or hands. This approach was both unhealthy and often unpleasant, though, and the wealthier gradually began using silk fabric instead. Italian adventurer

Marco Polo told us in the 13th century how servants in the courtyard of the Yuan dynasty had to shield their nose and ears with a silk and gold film cloth while serving food for the emperor.

The operational masks currently in use are Western imports. The use of masks in medical procedures dates at least back to 1897 but was not widely adopted until the beginning of the 20th century by the Chinese medical community.

At the end of 1910, famous Malaysian and Chinese doctor Wu Lien-Teh worked as the chief health officer in China when a northeastern China outbreak broke out. In the affected areas, Wu deepened his focus on prevention and control and soon defined the disease as a type of pneumonic plague that spread by droplets in the air. In addition to implementing now recognized measures — including quarantine patients and cordoning several towns — Wu also developed and patented an inexpensive facial sanitary mask providing some protection against the disease. It is a large-scale surgical gauze rolled into a 4-by-6 "piece of cotton that can be wrapped and tied in a knot. Quick and easy to make, almost anyone could afford it.

Throughout the 20th century, Chinese doctors and nurses continued to use Wu's style, enhancing it both here and there without making any major improvements. The then Chinese Food and Drug Administration discontinued Wu's mask in favor of older, more effective ones until the outbreak of SARS in 2004, which affected several hundred medical workers and revealed the shortcomings of the standard cotton mask.

But medical professionals are not the only Chinese to wear face masks regularly. Wave upon wave of cholera, smallpox, Diptheria, typhoid, scarlet fever, measles, malaria and dysentery were encountered in China during the Republican era (1912-1949). Around 1912 and 1948, Shanghai saw 12 outbreaks of cholera, six of which were significant. For 1938 alone, 11,365 cases were reported in the town, and 2,246 died.

One of the easiest and cheapest means of preventing these outbreaks in the world has been to make people wear masks.

Huang Wei, a librarian, One of the easiest and cheapest ways to prevent such outbreaks was for people to wear masks for the health authorities in that region. In 1929, the government responded to an epidemic of meningitis that started in Shanghai and then spread across the world by urging people to give masks and prevent public gatherings. In China's capital at the time, Nanjing Drum Tower Hospital sold facial masks to civil servants and ordinary citizens alike. In small towns such as Pinghu in the eastern province of Zhejiang, people are able to pick face masks.

Face masks were marketed as fashion accessories to facilitate their use in cosmopolitan Shanghai. In response to the outbreak of meningitis, prominent journalist Yan Duche addressed the value of masking in a 1929 column for Xinwen Bao newspaper entitled "The Most Trendy Fashionable Spring Accessory: A Black Face Mask" where he recommended that drugstores set aside profits and sell items required to prevent the outbreak, including masks, at a discount.

The government also suggested hiring famous celebrities and socialites for spring fashion shows to wear masks to encourage mainstream acceptance. Contemporary magazines often showed women in masks to be good hygiene symbols, making their covers into a status symbol for membership in the educated upper crust of the region. Certain sources created videos, in which housewives were taught how to knit wool masks in winter.

Woman: "Dear, why do you wear today, a face mask? Is this for control of epidemics? "One:" No! It is to remove the everlasting kisses. "Found in the journal" Manhua Jie Everything, "published in 1936. From the Shanghai Library, face masks became necessary defense from chemical and biological weapons with the onset of the Second Chinese and Japanese War in 1937. Magazines such as the China Newspaper Red Cross, the Air Defense Weekly, and the Student Magazine have started publishing articles on how to strengthen face masks by using gauze in neurotrophin, sodium carbonate and ammonium thioate additives, which are meant to be a poison gas safe mixture.

There is contradictory data as to whether masks — including high-tech versions such as the N95 — have security from C-19. But in the last century, China depended on face masks to protect it against cancer, chemical warfare and pollution. We may need to do that again in the absence of better options.

Chapter 1: Importance of Medical Face Mask

Why is it important to wear a mask, even if you do not have any symptoms? There are different opinions on whether you should be wearing a mask in public or not. Some health expert stated that there is no need to wear a mask if you do not present any symptoms, since this could limit the supplies needed in hospitals for healthcare personnel even more. Health authorities, in some parts of Asia, are constantly encouraging everyone to wear masks in public regardless wither they have symptoms, in order to prevent the spread of the virus and thus minimize its effects. A health expert at the University of Birmingham, KK Cheng, stated that "This is not to protect yourself but to protect people against the droplets that are coming out of your respiratory tract". To prevent the spread of the virus, Cheng also confirmed that it is extremely important that everyone follows the rule of social distancing and encourages everyone to stay at home as much as possible. It is very easy to get infected even if you are not coughing or sneezing; it is enough to get infected when people speak and breathe (droplets are still coming out). While performing randomized controlled trials that focused on other viruses, it was found that wearing a mask in public does not decrease infections. However, this studies had small sample sizes and in some of them not all participants wore face masks. Regarding on which type of mask is more appropriate to use, both surgical masks and the more protective N95 have shown to prevent respiratory

infections in healthcare personnel; but there has been a debate on which one is better to prevent any respiratory infection in patient care. An epidemiologist at the University of

Hong Kong stated that "when it comes to prevent infection, masks could work better at hospitals than in public; this is because healthcare personnel apply additional and important safety measures, such as hand-washing; but also because they are properly instructed on how to wear them." The great benefit of wearing masks in public comes from covering

mouths of people already infected. People that are ill or feel they start having symptoms of the current virus should not go out at all, but the biggest problem is that people that might

not experience any symptoms could also transmit the virus without knowing they are infected. This is why the shortage of face masks has pushed some individuals to produce their own cloth mask (including some retail shops as well). At the moment, studies that compare cloth masks to surgical masks are lacking.

Viruses and disease are often spread through germs that can survive in the air, outside of the host's body. These germs are made air-born and left on surfaces. This is done in several ways but one of the most likely scenarios is someone with a disease or virus sneezed or coughed. Disease is often spread through droplets. These droplets are exposed to the air and others through sneezing and coughing. In some cases, some breathing on you can infect you with droplets.

These droplets are so tiny we cannot see them without a microscope. Infection through droplets is the most common spread of disease and it's not hard to see why. When someone sneezes without covering their mouth the droplets from their sneeze can travel through the air for up to 6 feet. Let's say someone who is sick with a virus but doesn't know it yet, as is the case with some current viruses, is boarding a crowded train car. They sneeze without covering their mouth. That sneeze will travel up to 6 feet within the crowded train car and the droplets will infect everybody in that train car. If anyone on that train car is wearing a medical face mask, then they won't be infected by the droplets. If the one who was sick and sneezed is wearing a medical face mask, then no one in the car would be infected by the droplets.

Another way droplets are spread is through touch. Even covering your mouth when you sneeze and cough isn't helpful, especially if you cover your mouth with your hand. If you sneeze or cough into your hand and touch something before washing your hands, then you have spread the droplets onto the object. This happens often with doorknobs and even products on the shelf in a shop. Then these droplets are transferred from that object onto someone else's hands. They then end up infecting themselves by touching their mouth, nose, or eyes, or they handle and eat food and drink before washing their hands.

Guidelines on Wearing a Protective Mask In Public and at Work

Together We Will Beat Coronavirus

These are simple ways to explain how important it is to wear a medical face mask during these sensitive times when disease is spreading through the world. Droplets are the main way viruses and diseases are spread. The current Covid-19 virus is just one of many viruses that have harmed the health of our world. It is important that we take matters into our own hands. We must work to prevent the spread of disease. To do this we must take the necessary measures like washing our hands regularly, using hand sanitizers when we can't wash our hands, set up healthy daily routines, and wear a medical face mask whether we are healthy or sick.

How Close is Close? Understanding Close Contact & How To Deal With It

The following are a few scenarios that would constitute as close contact when thinking about contracting a virus.

Having direct contact with:

A person who has had direct physical contact with someone confirmed or suspected to have the virus (for example handshake);

A person who lives in a similar house as someone confirmed or suspected to have the virus;

A person who has had direct (eye to eye) contact with an instance of a virus, (under 2 meters and enduring longer than 15 minutes);

A person who has had unprotected direct contact with the emissions of someone confirmed or suspected to have the virus (for example contacting utilized paper cloths with uncovered hands);

A person who has been in a shut domain (for example homeroom, meeting room, emergency clinic sitting area) with an instance of a virus for in any event 15 minutes, a way off of under 2 meters;

A medicinal services proficient or other individual giving direct help to a case or research center workforce taking care of tests of someone confirmed or suspected to have the virus without the utilization of suggested PPE or by the utilization of unsatisfactory PPE;

A person who has traveled recently via an airplane in the two adjoining seats, or cruise toward any path, of someone confirmed or suspected to have the virus, their voyaging allies or parental figures and team individuals in the area of the airplane where the record case was situated.

The epidemiological connection may have happened inside a time of 14 days prior or after the event of the ailment for the situation being referred to.

What to Do if You Believe You Have Come in Contact with Someone with The Virus?

If you believe that you may have crossed paths with someone who has been confirmed to have the virus DO NOT PANIC! Instead try to separate yourself from the people around you and inform them so that they can take the necessary precautions in your household while you contact a medical professional for steps to go forward.

Who Is in Danger of Contracting the Virus?

In short, everyone stands the possibility of contracting the disease. This possibility, however, lessens if you follow the guidelines laid out by your local health department.

On the other hand, your changes of counteracting with the virus increases if you are constantly visiting public places or participate in large social events. This does, unfortunately, include those of us who are unable to work from home and are still venturing out on a daily basis.

People who live or have need to venture into areas that has been tagged as danger zones due to confirmed cases of the virus. These areas were labeled as such due to the plain fact that people who have been in close contact with an affirmed or plausible instance of a virus frequent these areas, making it easier for you to become infected.

Children, the elderly and persons known to have weaker immune systems are considered as high-risk groups. This means that they are in danger of contracting the virus easier and may have a harder time to fight off the virus.

So, Does This Mean that Doctors, Nurses, and Healthcare Professionals Are High Risk?

The ugly truth is that our fearless healthcare professionals come into contact with infected patients on a daily basis. Does this mean that they are all in danger of contracting the virus? In short, yes.

However, most, if not all, medical offices/centers should be equipped with the necessary protective gears required to limit the spread of the virus. Our healthcare professionals have also been trained to deal with such cases and as such would be better equipped to protect themselves against the virus.

Chapter 2: Technical Indicators of a Good Face Mask

It has been recommended by the CDC that people working in the health departments and others who are expected to socialize with infected patients to utilize N95 masks. All these are a sort of respirator mask which fits snugly into the facial skin and also made to filter small particles out of the atmosphere. When a breathing apparatus includes an"N95" designation, then so it can filter 95% of contaminants as small as 0.3 microns from the atmosphere. The viruses at the virus family are quite large (at least virus standards), and an average of they're just a little over 0.1 microns. Therefore, technically, despite an N95 mask, several virus contaminations may get through.

Additionally, it is essential to be aware that N95 masks do not function well for people or children who have hair on your face, and those who have lung problems may find it more difficult to breathe if wearing these masks. N95 masks can be known as a medical apparatus and also governed by the

U.S. Food and Drug Administration. It is possible to see a set of sterile masks.

You could find people wearing surgical masks, even those sterile paper masks which tug behind the ears. Regrettably, those masks are usually overly loose to necessarily work in preventing the focusing on virus patients. There remain a few things which you could do to safeguard your quality of life: wash your hands regularly (and wash them with heated soap and water), avoid touching your face or rubbing your mind, cook most your meal thoroughly and get sufficient sleep, and be sure that you're eating healthy and avoid anybody who's supposed to become sick with the virus (ostensibly, all what your mom always told you to accomplish).

Chapter 3: How to Properly Wear a Face Mask

It's important that the mask is work properly to ensure it is effective in protecting you against airborne droplets that may contain the coronavirus.

The following are the key points of how to properly wear a face mask:

Before touching your mask, clean your hands thoroughly with an alcohol-based sanitizer, or wash your hands soap and warm water for longer than 20 seconds.

Inspect the mask to make sure it is correctly folded, is clean and there are no holes.

Try not to touch the mask while using it. If you do need to touch the mask, ensure you clean your hands with soap and water of alcohol-based sanitizer.

If the mask becomes damp, or you are constantly sneezing and coughing into it, replace it with a new mask as soon as possible.

To remove the mask, remove it from behind by holding the ear straps of the elastic strap.

For a single use mask, discard it immediately in a closed bin then clean your hands with soap and water or an alcohol-based sanitizer.

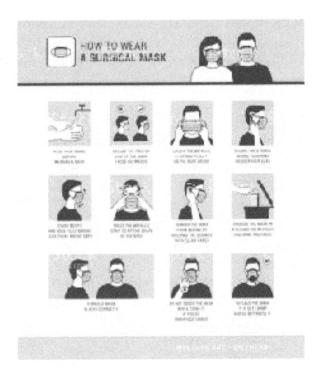

For masks that can be reused, such as the mask in this eBook, place it in the wash and wash it with a hospital grade disinfectant detergent.

Chapter 4: Types of Face Mask

Surgical Masks:

These are the most common masks that you see around, in the news, on the faces of people are mostly surgical face masks. Doctors, dentists and nurses often use this while treating their patients, mainly because these protect them from getting germs. Surgical masks can protect others from a patient suffering from any infectious disease. If any patient is wearing a surgical mask, and he coughs or sneezes, the mask doesn't allow the droplets to escape in the air around. But on the other hand, it doesn't protect you from getting infection if you are healthy. That's why health experts suggest that a surgical face mask should be worn by patients, not healthy people.

These masks are relatively thin and loose-fitted. The tiny droplets that come out with cough and sneeze (known as bio aerosols) containing the disease causing microbes are even tinier than the pores of this surgical mask and these droplets can seep through the parts of the mask. So, whereas they are helpful in stopping pathogens to escape if a patient wears them, they can't fully protect you if you are healthy and you face a patient with infectious disease who is not wearing it. In this way, surgical face masks are not a way of protection for healthy people.

In a nutshell, these masks are advisable to wear by the sick people to prevent spreading the disease.

Surgical face masks are disposable and are advised to use one time only.

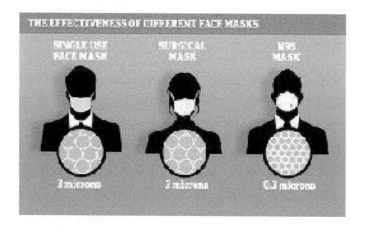

N95 Respirators:

Doctors and nurses who treat patients infected with any infectious disease use respirators. These are the same respirators which the construction workers use to protect themselves at work site. These respirators are heavy duty and designed to cover the face fully. They are air tight and can help you protect from getting infected to at least 95%. They can fit over your nose and mouth. CDC claims that these respirators, if worn properly, can filter out about 95% of particles and microorganisms those can use air as medium to travel. However, these respirators are not able to filter vapors, toxic gases and smoke. Yet, they are not full secure as they may allow 5% of particles to pass through which may cause infection. But 5% is a rare chance and though they can't promise a hundred percent protection, but a little precaution is much better than having no protection at all.

N95 masks can easily filter particles which are less than 0.3 micrometers. They are designed to filter particles like fumes, dust, aerosols, mists and smoke. They also can protect you against biological particles like pollen, animal dander, allergens, mold spores, and microorganisms. You can trust these respirators for protection against aerosol particles like cough or sneeze droplets that you can't see with your naked eyes.

Though they have a few limitations, for example, they do not fit on the little faces of children. If you have beards, long mustachios, or stubble, these respirators will not fit properly and protection will be compromised.

It is always advisable to practice wearing these respirators beforehand because a first time user may face difficulties in wearing them. A prior practice will prepare you to use them properly in the time of emergency.

P100 Respirator:

These are also known as gas mask. You can reuse them. These masks are designed to protect people involved in woodworking, those who face exposure to lead, solvents, asbestos and chemicals. They are considered the safest mode of protection, filtering out all oil and non-oil particles to 97.99%.

Full Face Respirators:

These respirators cover your full face. These can protect you from gases and vapors. These not only protects you from inhaling the particles of gases or vapor but also protect them entering your eyes. You can reuse them. Though these respirators are much safer than all N, P, R respirators, these are very costly and therefore, it is not in the range of common people.

Self-contained breathing apparatuses:

Basically, these are the most advanced type of face masks. They not only cover your whole face, but also have a breathing apparatuses with them. These help fire-fighters while they are on a mission to put out fire. These mask save them from dangerously polluted air.

Chapter 5: Precaution for The Usage of Medical Face Mask

There is no evidence to prove the effectiveness of various measures, such as cleaning and disinfection of masks.

When purchasing and using medical surgical masks, they must be purchased from regular hospitals and pharmacies. At the same time, the outer packaging of the product must have the production batch number, date of production, and period of use. Information such as production license, product registration number, and detailed product use instructions;

Always check if the packaging is undamaged before use, confirm the external packaging mark, production date, expiration date, and use it within the sterilization period;

It should be ensured that the mask is covered with the bridge of the nose to the jaw after deployment to obtain the expected protective effect;

Disposable medical surgical masks are prohibited from repeated use it;

Use with caution to those who are allergic to nonwovens

Medical-surgical masks should be handled in accordance with the requirements of hospitals and environmental protection departments after use.

Know How Masks Are Classified and Rated

N95 respirators, which have been reviewed, tested, and certified by the National Institute for Occupational Safety and Health (NIOSH), are typically the top quality masks recommended for use in dental environments. N95 breathers filter at least 95% of the contaminants in the air and are forbidden for use in patients with or suspected of respiratory illness. Nevertheless, most dental procedures do not need N95 respirators, but maybe in medical therapy-diagnosis with adequate triages should be deferred until later on after patients have sufficiently stabilized from signs of respiratory diseases.

The American Society for Research and Materials (ASTM) sets standards of consistency and the components that are most commonly used in dental conditions of the face masks. The standards measure fluid resistance, performance in bacterial filtration, submicron particulate filtration performance, differential pressure and flame propagation. Each mask earns a ranking according to its level of safety, in compliance with the ASTM standards.

The ASTM evaluations are optional, but they are carried out by the top dental mask manufacturers. The ASTM F2100-11 specification includes a graphical representation of the mask output rating on the package.

Watch for packaging saying anything like "grade 2" may mean that the manufacturer did not personally check the masks.

Wear Your Mask Right-Side-Up and Right-Side-Out

A dental mask should have three layers: the outer layer is moisture resistant, the middle layer cleans, and the inner layer covers the nose. The textures inside and outside are not identical.

Dental practitioners wear their masks more inside than you might expect. If the masks are color-coded, the contrast between the inside and the outside is easy to see. Review the manufacturer's instructions for non-color-coded masks. Furthermore, manufacturers usually pack their masks face up with the outside.

Dental facial masks should suit the face's contours. Laps between your skin and a mask's edge can allow pollutants to enter. Your face mask must be focused on correctly.

Like a waterfall, the flaps on a face mask will face down.

A face mask may offer extra protection against sickness. The CDC advises, however, that you use masks only if you are advised by a doctor or if you have respiratory symptoms, like COVID-19, to prevent infection for others around you. There are no known threats beyond the expense of purchasing these products.

Don (Put On) Your Mask Correctly

Some people make the error as they place their masks over their heads first. But before you securing your mask, make a small indentation or divot on your nose piece with your thumb. It helps better to place the mask on the bridge of the nose.

Open it a bit when you donate the mask (but not so much that the folds flicker). It makes the mask a perfect fit.

Then stretch the mask around the mouth and chin full. If you have a Stable Fit TM mask, change the bottom chin strap. This secures the exterior edges of the mask around the face and offers 360 degrees of security.

Often, practitioners with a broader face structure find like their masks are not adequately secure. They shorten the ear loops to compensate by making them into figure eight.

The concern is that the mask material is held up to the mouth and nose. Breath condensation travels inside the mask and allows the fibers of the mask material to swell in a process called wicking. In effect, this weakens the mask's ability to trap microbes. Using a Safe Fit mask is the best fit.

Take Off Your Mask Correctly

Much when there is a way to put on a face mask, there is a way to remove one. Incorrect removal of a tooth mask may lead to cross-contamination. Remember that the exterior surface of a face mask is coated with a film of aerosols, bacteria, blood bleeding and saliva.

Place your fingertips under each ear loop above your ear lobes to make a face mask and pull straight back.

Then remove the mask from the forehead and wash it. Should not contact the mask and use a mask even in the treatment room. Wash or using alcoholic hand rub shortly after the removal of the mask.

Although masks seem to be promising, other prevention steps are also necessary. Make sure you always wash your hands — especially if you are with people who may be ill. Make sure that the yearly influenza shot prevents you and others from transmitting the infection.

Chapter 6: Causes and Common Respiratory Problems

Not using respiratory masks and therefore inhaling some of the substances described above can cause serious problems. First, as a preliminary effect, it may be common for your nose or throat to become irritated. Such symptoms give mucus and irritation to the upper respiratory tract.

Secondly, not protecting your airways with PPE protective equipment can give you bronchitis, flu-like symptoms, a cold, or even asthma. It is important to know that when a worker develops breathing problems, cough, fever, muscle aches or general discomfort between four and six hours after being exposed to the substance, and these recur, we will undoubtedly be facing a key symptom of that your "illness" may be related to your job. Do not forget that the best solution is prevention and even more so in respiratory protection issues.

It is also relevant to strongly advise workers who are exposed to carbon dust, asbestos, or silica for more than 20 years since they can produce the disease known as emphysema.

Main causes of common respiratory problems of not using adequate protection

There are respiratory hazards during the workday, such as inhalation of dust, fumes, gases, vapors, or mists.

Some of these risks can end up being a respiratory disease Some of the substances that are in the air, and that can cause problems in the immediate future are:

Aerosol gases, especially malignant to painters who work on punctures, varnishes or lacquers. At this point, it is also advisable to notify hairdressers that they use hair fixatives, in lacquers, or similar gases, every day.

In short, the use of disposable masks has a direct impact on the health of the user, does not under any circumstances prevent working with full efficiency, nor does it represent a high economic burden in terms of price and durability, of course, it prevents long-term damage and advises asking for information before buying any mask to ensure good and correct protection.

How to Protect Yourself from Infectious Diseases & Live a Healthy Lifestyle

The current virus that we are battling across the world first appeared in the Hubei Province of China. To date, there have currently been 213,617 cases identified (this number is currently multiplying by the hour), and a whopping 8,791 deaths.

The silver lining in all this is that so far there have also been 84,314 people that have successfully recovered and we are hoping that that number will continue to grow in the coming months.

This can only happen, however, if we all do our part by ensuring we take the steps advised to practice good hygiene and to use the necessary protective gears.

Should You Wear a Mask and What is The Best Masks to Wear When Available?

The best answer I could provide to that would be that you should wear a mask whenever needed. For those who do not already have the virus it is solely a matter of preference. It is important to note that the act of wearing a mask will not guarantee that you won't contract a virus, but you will be protected from placing your hand in your mouth or nose.

It has been recommended, however, that all who suspect that they may have already come in contact with the virus to wear a protective mask in the event that it is unavoidable for you to come in contact with another person. This is especially true when around children, people with underlying health conditions or the elderly as the virus affects these groups significantly more.

Some folks go as far as recommending that a mask be worn regardless of if you suspect you have the virus or not as it is possible for you to have been affected but be unaware as the symptoms can take a while to show up. It can also be hard to differentiate if what you have is the common flu or something more serious.

Therefore, if you reside in a place where there has already been a particular virus instance, or even folks around you've got the flu, then you might choose to put on a mask for the reassurance. (Additionally, obtain a flu shot when you've not yet.)

Even though it is perhaps not being rigorously recognized this publication virus spreads are airborne and will disperse through tiny droplets expelled whenever somebody coughs or sneezes. All these droplets may also linger on surfaces and hitch a ride into the lymph nodes when someone rolls them after which brings their hands into their mouth or nose.

Chapter 7: How to Make Your Homemade Face Mask

As the Virus pandemic continuing to spread, it's now time for good people to start wearing a mask better than any mask.

You can't find a mask if you are like other Americans — at least not one at a fair price. And we'll teach you how to make your own.

But first, if you're puzzled with the post, "Whether I wear a mask or not," you're not alone.

The position of the Centers for Disease Control and Prevention has been strong since the start of the outbreak of Virus: safety masks are not mandatory for healthy people who do not work in the health care sector and do not care for an infected person at home.

However, many question the role of the CDC on masks as the death toll rises.

Dr. Anthony Fauci, director of the National Institute of Allergies and Infectious Diseases, told CNN on Tuesday that the Task Force on Cvirus in the White

House was considering suggesting the community-wide use of masks.

"Mitigation is the solution," Fauci said later in a White House press conference.

When pressed by journalists, President Trump proposed wearing a scarf instead of scarce shop masks. "We make millions of masks, but we want them to go to the hospitals," said Trump. On Wednesday, Mayor Eric Garcetti of Los Angeles urged everyone to wear home-made face masks when doing main tasks such as food shops and civil health officers in California to reduce the transmission of C-19 cloth face coating.

"Face-clothes are no substitute for physical drift or regular washing of hands, which we know is one of the most successful ways of reducing C-19 dissemination," said Dr. Sonia Angell, Director of the California Public Health Department. 'If wear a cloth face cover, it could also serve as a reminder for others to remain distant, helping reduce the spread of infectious particles by those who could be infected but do not have symptoms.' Given the lack of facial masks in the medical profession, it is important for us who cannot buy masks of our own as many of us don't even know how to sew or don't have access to the sewing supplies, no sewing DIY face masks are the best choice.

A Little Background On DIY Face Masks For Cvirus

Two types of facial masks can help reduce the risk of Cvirus: N95 masks that are tight and medical in grade and surgical facial masks — the masks described in the tutorials below — that are relatively thin and lose fitting.

An analysis of SmartAirFilters.com's home-made face masks revealed that the cotton T-shirts and cotton pillowcases are the best material at home to make DIY facial masks based on their ability to absorb particles but remain breathable.

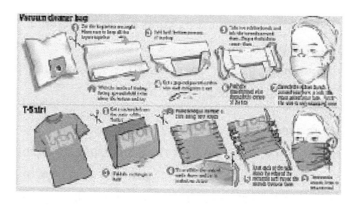

And of course, follow all your local protocols and avoid leaving the house unless it is necessary.

Make Your Own Face Mask—No Sewing Machine Required

You already have what you need at home.

Let's be clear about this: masks are not guaranteed to protect you from C-19, however successful.

"A mask is always just as good as the wearer and is not a replacement for a social distance and good grooming of hands," says Anna Davies, one of the England public health researchers.

In an ideal world, everyone would wear their own masks in public to prevent the virus from spreading secretly, and the CDC will be considering suggesting that everyone, not just those with symptoms, wear masks officially.

Unfortunately, masks are a little difficult to come across now, with the procurement of masks raising the availability of health workers who need them. Even if the CDC makes no new guidelines, anyone who cares for a sick lover certainly would have at least two to sterilize the one while wearing the other.

Our tutorial is a simple project for people who have no sewing machine, adapted by Helpful Engineering from MakerMask for a global C-19 open-source project. Although many of the projects call for cotton, Davies says that there is no evidence that it is better or worse than other fabrics, that it is comfortable and suitable for people. Due to researchers 'hypothesis about the hydrophilic (water-) qualities of cotton masks, which lead to higher rates of respiratory infection, MakerMask suggested we use a synthetic hydrophobic material similar (not identical) to that used in surgical masks. So even people in their own homes have it right.

Stats

Time: 90 minutes if sewn by hand

Estimated materials cost: less than $5

Difficulty: medium

Tools

Needle and thread

Scissors

Ruler

Clothing iron

Sewing or safety pins

Permanent marker

(Optional) Seam ripper

Materials

1 medium non-, ribbon- polypropylene bag with

2 pipe- (or plastic- pulling twists)

(Optional) 60 inches, 1/2 to 1-inch long.

Instructions

You already have everything you intend to do at home.

1. Clean your reusable food bag.

Caution: we suggest explicitly a reusable non-woven polypropylene food bag (NWPP for short), not a disposable unwrappable bag. It might sound obvious, but you'll have to breathe through the mask. Stay away from isolated bags (usually with some foil on the inside) or insulated bags with plastic lining.

Note: If possible, choose the bag you will find with the longest handles. This project is better if you can use it as mask belts. If the handles are inadequate, we'll explain how to make ribbon belts.

2. Cut the sides off the food bag to keep the packaging flat. Do not cut off handles. Do not cut off the handles.

3. Break the material into two parts. Cut it off just as you do the side seams when your bag has a seam at the bottom. You will receive two clean NWPP sheets, each with its own handle.

4. Measure and cut a sheet of paper. Measure the edge with the handle to reach the middle with your ruler. Label your permanent marker for it. As a starting point, measure 4 1/2 inches back to the handles, and mark again. Measure 9 inches from each mark and draw vertical cutting lines parallel. Link the bottom lines. You will have a 9-by-9-inch

square with the handle on the top with a finished (sewn) bottom.

Remark: If your handle is too large to fit inside the measured rectangle, it is easy to skip Step 8 and use the ribbon instead (Step 9).

5. Repeat step 4 on the other content layer.

6. Fold over each handle on the opposite edge. Put up one plate with the incorrect side (former interior of the bag) and fold half an inch of material in from that bottom. Iron the fold to set it on low heat. Then add it to the bottom for a quarter inch. Place the other sheet on the right side (former exterior bag), and fold it in a half-, iron, like the other sheet, and sew it in from the edge a quarter-.

Warning: polypropylene is a plastic form. It will melt with a high wind; destroy your project, and, most likely, your iron. If there are no "poly" configurations, seek the lowest one (typically silk) and slightly increase it if the fold is not set.

7. Set the sheets together. Your mask is going to have two cloth layers. Place the handle facing the left on one of the sheets on your work surface. Place the other with the handle facing right on top of it. Place in place. Lock in place.

Note: The printed side of the sheets should be oriented in the same direction so that the mask's back is different from the front. Davies claims this will help to ensure that you don't confuse the mask with your dirty mouth and nose.

8. Make head ties. Place the handles in half and cut them in the middle. Keep your face balanced with the handles from the arms, and see to it that the handles are long enough to spare you at least 4 inches on the back of your head.

9. (Optional) Render ribbon belts. If your handles are not long enough to transform into braces, you will have to make it your own. Cut the ribbons and pin where the handles once were. Test the fit with the mask. If the ribbon length is right, double the thread and stitch the parts on the wrong side of the boards.

10. Sew together the boards. Double the thread and tie all the edges.

11. Full the bottom lip. Like you did in step 6, fold it in half an inch and iron it to the rim. Sew it closed the bottom for a quarter-inch.

12. Render the noseband flexible. Again, fold over and iron it about half an inch from the top edge.

Switch the pipe cleaners together or twist ties and cut them to the same width as the mask. Fold to break them at their ends. Tuck in the fold the metal links and secure the fold-over them. Then sew the fold underneath and on the sides of the links to protect them. Create three folds for the expansion of the mask. Pleats will have an outer diameter of around 1 1/2 inches, an inner one-half inch running parallel to the nose line. Draw lines on your cloth if it works, fold them, then iron them. Bring them in line by stitching a quarter inch on both sides of the lip. Double the stitch this time to make sure the seam is tight.

13. Sterilize your body. Sterilize your mouth. Take your mask in boiling water for 10 minutes before using it for the first time. Repeat this step between applications.

Chapter 8: Materials For Making Homemade Face Mask

We want to introduce to you exciting research where the Researchers selected a range of household materials useful for homemade masks and tested the capacity to capture virus-sized particles in comparison to a surgical mask.

The test was performed to see how well those different materials coped with selected bacteria and viruses. For this research, the researcher decided 2 pathogens:

-        the Bacillus atrophaeus bacteria (0.93-1.25 microns in size),

-        the Bacteriophage MS2 virus (0.023 microns in size).

In this research, the selected materials Vs. a surgical mask is the follows:

-        Vacuum cleaner Bag

-        Tea Towel

-        Cotton Mix

- Cotton T-Shirt 100%

- Antimicrobial Pillow

- Scarf

- Pillowcase

- Linen

- Silk

The question is: can homemade masks capture smaller viruses?

To answer this question, we select the test vs. Bacteriophage MS2 particles that 0.02 micron, which is 5 times smaller than the common Virus.

The Vacuum cleaner Bag and a Double layer of tea Towels have a filter capacity close to a Surgery Mask, how conformable and how easy it breathing wearing A Vacuum cleaner bag or 2 tea towel layers mask: the comfortability depend by the time you will wear them, and the breathability it is not easy!

When it comes to protecting yourself from bacteria, there is never enough methods that will keep you safe. Wearing a face mask is just never enough. Bacteria is detrimental to health and can spread quickly. Good hand hygiene practice is necessary at this point. Since microbes and germs stays in the hand, it is essential that you keep it clean at all times. Washing hands with soap and water or with a hand sanitizer, together with putting on a medical face mask is an effective combination in combating bacteria.

Not all bacteria are harmful. Some bacteria in the intestine like Lactobacillus acidophilus helps in the digestion of food and destroys disease-causing organisms. Washing your hands is simple. However, if you don't wash it the correct way, there is a possibility that some germs are still lingering in one part of your hand. Follow these simple steps to wash your hands effectively with soap and water.

• Wet your hands with clean running water. Turn the tap off and apply soap.

• Rub your hands together with the soap until it forms lather. Lather the backs of your hands, in-between the fingers, and under the

nails. Make sure you lather all parts of your hands.

• Scrub your hands like that between 15 - 20 seconds.

● Once you are done scrubbing, rinse your hands well under the running water.

Dry your hands with a clean towel.

In the absence of soap and water, you can use alcohol-based hand sanitizer. Alcohol-based sanitizers are not 100% effective against certain germs and harmful chemicals like pesticides. However, they are good alternatives to handwashing. In case you don't know how to wash your hands with a sanitizer, follow these simple steps.

● Ensure your hands are visibly dry.

● Apply the recommended amount in one palm and rub it together with the other.

● Rub in-between the fingers and make sure your entire hands are well covered.

Once skin is dry, stop rubbing the sanitizer. Always put hand sanitizer in your bag because soap and water are not always available. This will keep you prepared for any eventuality. While you may think that washing hands and wearing a face mask are two vital ways of protecting yourself from bacteria, there are other couple of ways you can also protect yourself from germs. Other ways of protecting yourself from bacteria include:

• Use Antibiotics - When you find out that you or your family is sick, consult a health practitioner for best antibiotics treatment. Although antibiotics are effective against harmful bacteria, they have some side effects. So if you experience one or two side effects as a result of using it, desist from taking it.

• Vaccination - One of the best line of body defense is the use of vaccines. A number of diseases and bacterial infections can be prevented by vaccination. While many vaccines are given in childhood, adults can also benefit from vaccinations.

Clean All Kitchen Utensils and Equipment - Kitchen hygiene is crucial in protecting you from bacteria. Eating unsafe food is one of the fastest way of contracting bacteria. So, you need to make sure that you prepare your food safely. Wash raw meat, fish, with salt. Clean utensils, tools, and kitchen counters.

• Practice Good Hygiene - Ensuring that you have all-round hygiene is critical. Make sure you wash your clothes and bed sheets all the time. Bacteria can hide in them for days and when you wear them without washing, you get infected. Bathe and brush your tooth for at least twice a day. Keep your environment clean. Clean all surfaces in the home, trim all tall grasses if you have any and empty the bins regularly. Bacterial can infest in all these and get transferred by the air to you.

• Drink Enough Water - Research has shown that drinking water after you are up in the morning will kickstart your body functions and prepare it for the day. Drinking enough water also helps to keep your skin smooth and prevent dryness. Drinking 2 - 3 liters of water per day will help boost the immune system and fight against bacteria.

Chapter 9: Advantage and Disadvantage of Homemade Face Mask

Advantages of Using Face Masks

A mask is a baggy, dispensable gadget that makes a physical obstruction between the wearer's mouth and nose and potential contaminants in the quick condition. Whenever worn appropriately, a mask is intended to help square enormous molecule beads, sprinkles, showers, or splatter that may contain infections and microorganisms, shielding it from arriving at the wearer's mouth and nose.

A mask may likewise help lessen the introduction of the wearer's salivation and respiratory emissions to others. Mask additionally remind wearers not to contact their mouth or nose, which could somehow or another exchange infections and microscopic organisms subsequent to having contacted a sullied surface.

A mask, by configuration, doesn't channel or little square particles noticeable all around that might be transmitted by hacks, wheezes, or certain clinical methods. Face mask additionally doesn't give total security from germs and different contaminants due to the free fit between the outside of the face mask and the face.

Assortment productivity of mask channels can go from under 10% to almost 90% for various makers' mask when estimated utilizing the test parameters for NIOSH accreditation. In any case, an investigation found that in any event, for face masks with "great" channels, 80–100% of subjects bombed an OSHA-acknowledged subjective fittest, and a quantitative test demonstrated 12–25% leakage.

The present-day mask is produced using paper or other non-woven material and ought to be disposed of after each utilization

A mask, or method mask, is planned to be worn by wellbeing experts during a medical procedure and certain human services procedures to get microorganisms shed in fluid beads and pressurized canned products from the wearer's mouth and nose.

Proof backings the adequacy of mask in lessening the danger of contamination among other social insurance laborers and in the community. In any case, a Cochrane audit found that there is no reasonable proof that dispensable face masks worn by individuals from the careful group would diminish the danger of twisted diseases after clean, careful procedures.

For medicinal services laborers, security rules suggest the wearing of a face-fit tried N95 or FFP3 respirator mask rather than a mask in the region of pandemic-influenza patients, to diminish the presentation of the wearer to possibly irresistible vaporizers and airborne fluid beads.

Network and home settings, the utilization of facemasks and respirators, for the most part, are not suggested, with different estimates favored, for example, evading close contact and keeping up great hand hygiene.

Mask is prevalently worn by the overall population lasting through the year in East Asian nations like China, Japan, South Korea and Taiwan to diminish the opportunity of spreading airborne maladies to other people, and to forestall the taking in of airborne residue particles made via air pollution.

In Japan and Taiwan, it is entirely expected to see these mask worn during the influenza season, as a demonstration of thought for other people and social responsibility. Mask gives some insurance against the spread of ailments, and extemporized masks give about half as much protection. A few nations like

Slovakia presented required masks in broad daylight transport and open spaces during the coronavirus pandemic in 2020.

All the more as of late, because of the rising issue of brown haze in South and Southeast Asia, masks and an air separating face mask are presently every now and again utilized in significant urban communities in India, Nepal and Thailand when air quality crumbles to dangerous levels. Furthermore, face masks are utilized in Indonesia, Malaysia, and Singapore during the Southeast Asian fog season.

Furthermore, the mask has become a design explanation, especially in contemporary East Asian culture supported by its ubiquity in Japanese and Korean mainstream society which bigly affect East Asian youth culture. Air sifting careful style masks are very well known across Asia, and accordingly, numerous organizations have discharged masks that not just forestall the taking in of airborne residue particles but, on the other hand, are fashionable. Mask with enlivening, structures are famous in nations in which they are worn in public.

Mask may likewise be worn to disguise character. In the US, banks, comfort stores, and so forth have prohibited their utilization because of hoodlums over and again doing as such. In the 2019–20 Hong Kong fights, some protestors wore face masks among different sorts of the mask to keep away from acknowledgment, and the administration attempted to boycott such utilize.

Benefits of Masks and How They Keep You and Others Safe

Lots of folks can wear facemasks that will help protect against hazardous or dust airborne contaminants -- especially when they live or work within an environment where contamination, chemicals, and allergies are trivial. During the influenza season, some could also decide to utilize masks to help block the transmission of viruses and bacteria.

For those who have a chronic disease, wearing a breathing apparatus can be particularly essential. Here Are Just Some of the primary reasons:

- People with chronic diseases might have increased sensitivities to allergens, dust or specific compounds and wear a mask to avoid inhaling these sores
- If you are a caregiver of someone having a compromised immune system, then you may wear a mask to help stop

yourself bypassing contamination on for a loved one.

- Facing a diminished or suppressed immune system due to your disease or drugs can make you vulnerable to having influenza or an infectious disease.
- Obtaining a cold or the flu when you have a chronic illness could aggravate your Present symptoms or create a Flare-up.

Research has indicated masks might well not be 100 percent effective in preventing the spread of potentially harmful airborne contaminants; however, they can help lessen the probability of contamination. You'll find two primary sorts of masks, facial masks, and respirators, even though they look like they will have some crucial differences.

Facemasks cover the mouth and nose but certainly are looser-fitting and do not seal completely. They made to described as a barrier contrary to droplets of fluid, like coughs or sneezes, which may contain viruses. However, they don't avoid the spread of airborne contamination. Some facemasks are disposable, while some may be cleaned and reused.

Respirators additionally work as a barrier. However, they believed more powerful than facial masks for avoiding the spread of germs because they produce an ideal seal (if correctly used) and filter 95 percent of airborne contaminants, both big and small.

A respirator might be used to protect against airborne contagious diseases and may likewise be utilized when handling hazardous substances. Some are manufactured for single usage while some are reusable and created using filler cartridges that have to replaced occasionally.

Deciding whether to employ a face mask or Respirator is dependent upon your wellbeing, individuals that you may come in contact with, and your surrounding ecosystem.

We desired to learn which brands of face masks and respirators people who have chronic disease find most reliable; therefore, we asked our Mighty community that masks that they wear to reduce their probability of becoming ill

Here are some recommendations about the Face Mask:

1. N95 Respirator

This disposable respirator can you to maintain reliable respiratory security of 95 percent filtration efficacy against individual non-oil established particles. The Cool Flow Exhalation Valve helps reduce heat buildup in the Respirator.

The N95 Respirator can be sourced at your local medical supply stores and at times even hardware stores, when available. Just be sure that the fit is very tight. The mask is frequently used in hospitals on patients confirmed to have contagious diseases.

2. Vog-mask

Vog-masks can be a filtering respirator designed for public usage, which may help protect you against allergens, inadequate quality of air, and also airborne contaminants. It could filter up to 99 percent of airborne particles.

4. Disposable Hospital Masks

These commercial-grade facial masks made for overall protective functions. They feature an aluminum shield you can mold to fit tightly across your nose.

Hospital-type masks are both disposable and delicate. We arrange them by circumstance. Each mask is merely good until it becomes moist --

significantly less than one hour. Shifting is essential in case you genuinely possess an immunocompromised condition.

5. K-pop Facemasks

These facemasks are completely cotton, are available in fun black-and-white layouts, and also help protect against airborne dust, germs, and allergens, smoke, contamination, pollen, and ash.

7. <u>Home Depot Neoprene Dust Mask</u>

This neoprene respirator created for outdoor or landscaping work. Nonetheless, it offers all-purpose protection and certainly will filtrate up to 99.9 percent of most particulates and dust. Its double valve exhaust offers one-way breathing, expels warmth, and maximizes temperature.

8. MyAir Face Mask

MyAir facemasks block 99.997 percentage of germs, bacteria, pollutants, and allergens. The reusable two-way mask sold with three replaceable filters also comprises high-level filtration technology, which will help reduce moisture loss.

9. Cambridge Mask Co.

Cambridge masks are reusable and washable. They could filter out nearly 100 percent of particulate matter, allergies or allergens, atmosphere contamination, and dangerous airborne pathogens such as germs and bacteria.

Disadvantages of Using Face Masks

If you want to create your masks for personal use, to give you peace of mind, there is nothing wrong with it. However, the important thing to understand is that stitching your face mask may not prevent you from getting an infection, especially if you are engaging in risky behavior, such as staying in crowded places or continuing to meet friends.

Since some infections appear to be asymptomatic but can be transmitted by someone who hosts the virus, it is essential for the health and well-being of those over 65 years of age and those with basic conditions to know what proven measures will help. to protect them as immune-deficient people and an elderly person should take extra measures as homemade face masks should not be relied on since it does not guarantee 100% protection and the survival rate for this category of persons is very low hence it's not worth the risk putting your trust on a homemade face mask while going outside, since the risk is far greater than the benefits.

HOMEMADE MASKS ARE NOT STERILIZED

Another difference between homemade masks and factory-made masks and factory-made masks concerns sterilization, which is very important in the hospital setting. With handmade facial masks, there is no guarantee that the mask is free from bacteria, viruses or other microbes - however, measures such as washing masks can help combat this.

Chapter 10: The Basics of Surgical Mask Selection

The problem of hospital infection prevention is a regular challenge for both health staff members and patients. Surgeons, anesthetists, nurses, and infection control professionals have educated views and individual convictions on the causes and avoidance of infection in the clinical setting. It has to be done to remove or at least reduce infection causative agents is a problem for all.

The history of surgery and the cap, dressing, and masking procedures dates back to the 1860s. Live microorganisms are thought to be extracted from the blood, bare skin, and mucus membranes. Studios by Tuneval in Great England suggested that the use of operational masks does not affect the number of possible pathogenic bacteria in the air near the site of the operation, and question the value of the use of surgical masks1. While there is no evidence to suggest that masks are not necessary for reducing wound infections, surgical masks are used in throughout recent years, the safety of the healthcare professional and the patient has become a question in infection control and is becoming increasingly complex. Some of the problems relating to the real need to wear an operating mask in the surgical area (OR) are controlled.

Transmission-based precautions are advised in the treatment of patients with highly transmissible or epidemiologically significant infections evidence or potential infection, or where specific measures other than standard measures are required.

Droplet precautions: a surgical mask is typically used to guard against large bacterial particles that are spread by direct contact, and can only move small distances (up to 3 feet) from coughing and sneezing sick patients. If prone individuals enter the rooms of patients confirmed or suspected of having measles (rubeola) or chickenpox, then respiratory security will be given to them.

FDA. FDA. Medical devices are governed by the Food and Drug Administration (FDA). Section 201(h) of the Federal Food, Drug and Cosmetic Act describes a medical product. The definition includes any article intended for use in human-made remedies, reduction, diagnosis, or prevention of disease that does not accomplish its intended purposes by means of chemical intervention or is based on metabolism (e.g., a medicinal substance).

An example of an item regulated as a medical device is a surgical mask.

NIOSH. NIOSH. NIOSH is a federal agency and branch of the Department of Health and Human Services, which identifies substances that pose potential health problems and recommends limits on exposure to OSHA. NIOSH carries out comprehensive protection, and health studies provide technical assistance and propose criteria for OSHA adoption. NIOSH also certifies ventilation gear.

Masks are often worn in the OR, where sterile supplies are delivered, in clean cores, and at scrub sinks. Whenever blood splashing, spray or aerosol, or other potentially contagious materials may be created, masks with face guards and masks and protective eyewear are required.

The healthcare staff typically wear a face mask to protect against the transmission of large-particle droplets produced in direct contact and usually only fly short distances (up to 3 feet) from sick patients who cough or sneeze. The OSHA Blood Borne Pathogen Standard (BBPS) (29 CFR 1910.1030) requires the use of goggles, eye scapes, and face covers under specific circumstances to reduce the risk of blood borne pathogens exposure. In December 1991, this regulation was released. The aim of BBPS is to remove or decrease worker access to blood borne pathogens such as hepatitis B (HBV) and HIV. This requires standardized protocols, risk preparation, patient screening, vaccine and medication standards, safety reviews, workplace conditions, identification, and personal protective equipment issued by employers. The BBPS:

Ø   Needs a mask used for eye shielding or a chin-length facial protector to be used while conditions for blood contact and other highly contagious body fluids or materials occur.

Ø   It requires a face mask to prevent the passage of blood or other infectious body fluids to the skin, eyes, mouth, or other mucous membranes of employees under regular splashing and spraying conditions.

Masks with different characteristics can be found in various forms and picked for personal security and design and fitness preferences. The most popular styles in the workroom are perfect tie-on, duckbill, cone-shaped, flat-folded with shields, and duckbill with shields. High fluid-resistant ear loop covers are also available that can be used by roaming nurses in the OR.

Masks are only successful if they are correctly worn. Masks minimize the flow from the wearer of infectious pieces to the atmosphere and help shield the wearer from splashing or splashing of blood and body fluid. Masks would be secure, protecting both the mouth and the nose. Workers in the sterile area should use a face mask or clear eyewear. The design will ensure that there is no tenting on the sides of the mouth to spread or encourage bacteria to enter. A narrow folding strip on the nose would match similarly. Masks should be periodically adjusted and damp at all moments. When the mask is removed, treat the strings only and immediately discharge them into a waste bin. This is not uncommon for masks to be put beneath the nose or moistened with blood or body fluids. A mask should never hang or peddle around the face, nor should it be folded and inserted in a pocket for later use.

Effectiveness of surgical masks

Few tests have demonstrated the efficacy of surgical masks for sterile field safety. The focus on the safety of the patient during the procedure in the production of operation masks to date has, therefore, been focused on filtering capacity and has been calculated in various ways (Belkin, 1997). The efficacy of mask filter aggregation is highly subjective. Tests have shown varying levels of penetration based on particle size and the research methods employed (Cooper et al., 1983b; Tuomi, 1985; Brosseau et al., 1997; McCullough et al., 1997; Willeke and Qian, 1998). Two reports suggest that the wearing of a mask has little effect on the occurrence of surgical wound infection (Orr, 1981; Tunevall, 1991). One research found that wearing masks under headgear inhibits the minimization of face seal leakage (Ha'eri and Wiley, 1980).

Non-Surgical Masks and Alternative Materials

In addition to FDA-approved medical masks, some look or tissue cotton masks are available. During the epidemic of Extreme Acute Respiratory Syndrome (SARS) in Asia, masks of this type were widely used (see Chapter 3). In fact, in emergency situations, staff and the public have sometimes covered their airways with ready-to-use items (such as sheets or towels) or with unapproved plastic facemasks, sold as respiratory aid in hardware shops.

New reusable surgical masks were made of woven fabric that only separated air from the surgical wound. In the early 1960s, surgical masks often made from cheesecloth were replaced with the synthetic materials mentioned previously, providing both increased filtration performance and bacterial filtration.

Specific mannequin research has shown that these fabrics can minimize aerosol particulate amounts and some water-soluble gasses and vapors at pressure decrease suitable to breathe in accident situations. In tandem with innovative facial fit methods (e.g., nylon hose), leaking can be minimized (Cooper et al. 1983b). The animal tests indicate that carefully designed six-layer gauze masks decrease the occurrence of tuberculosis bacilli infection by 90% to 95% (Lurie and Abramson 1949). Regulatory standards ensure, however, that a mask does not allow blood or other potentially contagious products, under usual operating circumstances and for the duration of time the protective equipment is being used, to move or touch the wearer's face, head, or mouth or other mucous membranes (OSHA, 1992).

Learn the pros and cons of using a diy face mask to help with acne_

Acne is one of the worst factors that can harm our skin and is not only limited to adolescents. Surprisingly, acne affects many people every day, and there is a full beauty industry that seeks to cure this condition, from facial masks to foundations. Naturally, different natural strategies can appear enticing to attempt to keep your face transparent, and one of these is to keep a facial mask. Like often, there are benefits and drawbacks of using acne natural facial masks. It used to be exclusive to the day spa has now come to our baths and daily rituals, and several different natural masks are available on the market. There is almost everything you can think of from charcoal to honey to cover your hair, and most of those things are natural.

You want to step back and examine your acne problem before deciding on a specific natural face mask; is it wrong? You may want to figure out whether the acne condition is caused by dry skin or even everyday dirt and grit. A mask does not do you any good if you will not take the other measures to exfoliate and cleanse your face, and that is why many therapies for counter acne fail. We will take a look at the benefits and drawbacks of using one of the different natural face masks to tackle the acne problem.

Pro: A Natural Face Mask Will Open Your Pores

One of the principal culprits behind acne is the obstruction of your pores. Whether it's dirt or oily skin, the outcome is still trapped, so you will want to cleanse your face many times daily. A decent washing mask opens your pores and extracts any debris from them, leaving your skin with a thoroughly cleaner feeling and look. Of course, using a face mask is not the only way you want to combat acne, but it can be a significant first step in the battle against clear skin.

Con: Overexposure Can Cause A Rash

Like most good things, too much good can cause you a problem, and the same can be said with the facial masks for time. You won't remove the face mask for long because prolonged exposure will create a bad skin rash. The skin rash is particularly a drawback if you attempt to combat acne in that way, and if you have a facial mask, it takes time to read the instructions, and following the time limits is an essential part of the proper application of the mask.

Pro: No Chemical Burns

There are some significant benefits when it comes to treating acne, and one of them is that you do not suffer any chemical burns. Many counter-acne remedies tend to flame the skin if they are not applied correctly, and that is sadly the path the acne industry has taken toward the full treatment of acne. Still, without risking a fire, a natural mask will cleanse your face and exfoliate your pores. The natural approach would be perfect if you love holistic beauty treatments and want to prevent rash for your face.

Con: A Natural Face Mask Might Not Work for All Acne Cases

Here's the thing, acne will have her own mind. The typical path does not even work with the most difficult situations or other forms of acne. Usually, this is when acne regulation comes into play, and there are several explanations that an acne case may be so serious. Hormones appear to make our skin split up very much and can cause acne levels to fluctuate on our skin, where there is a hormone imbalance. While this is unpleasant, there won't be too many appropriate natural solutions for this.

Acne Can Be Controlled with The Right Mixture of Treatments

Perhaps nothing that is so physically and mentally fragile as acne, because your beauty is such an essential part of your self-esteem. It can be a difficult battle to get your acne under control, and often the counter-remedies are either not an effective option or are just too strong. A natural face mask may be a far more effective option, if you are tired of the drying out of your face, to help keep your skin tall and potentially remove your acne problem in a much more enjoyable manner.

Considerations in The Use of Homemade Masks to Protect Against COVID-19

Homemade masks may include those that are:

ü   Made of linen, cotton, for example.

ü   Attach other masks or filters into pockets.

ü   Be worn on breathers N95 (in an effort to reuse breathable).

Homemade masks are not medical appliances and are thus not regulated, such as surgical masks and respirators. There are a number of drawbacks to their use:

ü　　　　　They have not been checked in compliance with recognized criteria.

ü　　　　　They cannot have complete protection against the particulate matter of virus size.

ü　　　　　The edges of the nose and mouth are not built to create a barrier.

ü　　　　　Bacteria are not similar to those found in surgical masks or respirators.

ü　　　　　They can be hard to breathe, though, and they can keep you from having the amount of oxygen your body needs.

ü　　　　　These will need regular modification, increase the touch of your hands with your face, and increase the risk of infection.

Such masks cannot be used to remove fragments of the infection that can be spread by coughing, sneezing, or other surgical procedures. They will not have complete protection against coronavirus due to their inherent loose fit and materials.

Just N95 operating breathable (not surgical masks) fit-tested NIOSH-approved are intended to offer maximum safety. Such respirators are Health Canada licensed medical equipment. An N95 respirator is a respiratory safety system designed for very near facial fit and extremely effective airborne particle filtration. The classification 'N95' indicates that the respirator blocks at least 95% of very small test particles in thorough research.

Medical masks are often medical devices that use materials that block at least 95% of very small test particles, but they do not fit tightly to the face so that the user is not fully shielded. To have extra protection, they must be used in conjunction with other personal protective equipment (PPEs).

Following the COVID-19 epidemic, Santé Canada received valuable guidance to improve the usage of masks and respirators.

The Guidelines on coronavirus prevention from the Public Health Agency of Canada include guidance on wearing masks if needed and include:

ü   If you are a good citizen, you cannot use a mask to avoid the spread of COVID-19.

ü   If you're not sick, wearing a mask will give you a false sense of comfort.

ü   There is a possible possibility of contamination by misuse and reuse of masks.

ü   They must also be updated regularly.

ü   Nevertheless, if you have signs of COVID-19 as you are receiving or waiting for treatment, your health care provider may consider wearing a mask. Masks are a good part of infection prevention and control procedures in this case. The mask is a foil that serves to prevent tiny droplets from scattering as you toast or sneeze.

Chapter 11: Mistakes While Using Face Mask

There are a lot of mistakes that we usually do while using a face mask; some of them are as follows.

Worn Incorrect

In the meantime, inadequate face masks flourish. The market in Hong Kong, for instance, is moderately unregulated, and the promoted cases of many face mask available to be purchased, particularly on the web, are expanded or inside and out bogus, yet the appeal of assurance against unnerving sicknesses like the coronavirus plays on human dread and opens up wallets. Therefore, numerous individuals wind up purchasing an inappropriate mask or wear a decent mask mistakenly, with exacerbated abuse possibly helping spread instead of forestalling perilous respiratory pathogens like COVID-19. Calm down with the wrong feeling that everything is fine, a mask wearing client may enter high-hazard territories, open themselves to more coronavirus threats and proceed to exponentially contaminate others.

Utilized masks are not discarded rapidly and properly. Utilized masks have development of conceivably irresistible particulates that could incorporate coronavirus and different pathogens, and whenever left around, they can cross-taint beforehand clean regions.

It is utilizing a fake face mask. The highest quality level for careful face masks is ASTM-F2100. However, there are numerous masks that appear to be comparative, made of modest materials that don't satisfy that guideline and don't give sufficient obstruction against malady. Just purchase from trustworthy vendors; face masks produced using inadequate material proliferate on the web.

Wearing a Mask for Too Long

Wellbeing authorities state you shouldn't be wearing defensive face masks as a safeguard measure against becoming ill. Truth be told, they state wearing a mask may make you bound to discover something.

Fears over the spreading coronavirus have prompted a monstrous lack of defensive face mask over the world with many trusting they can forestall the ailment by wearing a mask.

The mask most normally found in regions influenced by the spread of COVID-19 is the face mask. Wellbeing authorities state this mask is intended to forestall the spread of germs by getting particles removed by wheezing or hacking. It isn't intended to keep solid individuals from becoming ill.

The face mask is not proposed to be utilized more than once. On the off chance that your mask is harmed or ruined, or if breathing through the mask gets troublesome, you should evacuate the face mask,

dispose of it securely, and supplant it with another one. To securely dispose of your mask, place it in a plastic sack and put it in the waste. Wash your hands after taking care of the pre-owned mask. Pulling it under the chin.

Masks Are Not Disposed Appropriately

As utilized face mask may convey germs including the coronavirus, they shouldn't be haphazardly disposed of as waste. Since the infection can get by for a couple of days in sticky conditions, the pre-owned masks may turn into another wellspring of contamination. On the off chance that the waste masks are hurled in a kept space, for example, a lift, they may defile the earth, representing a potential danger to individuals inside it. Likewise, it is unseemly to blend sullied mask in with family unit squander.

Given the trash arranging is presently actualized in just a couple of urban communities, blended waste normally exists. The blend of the contaminated mask and recyclable waste may make a potential peril refuse authority when they put delivers the waste receptacles to gather recyclable things. More terrible, in the event that somebody just tosses a pre-owned mask in the city, somebody may get it, or awful attempt to gather them to sell second-hand.

In this manner, it is vital for the administration to urge individuals to ensure the pre-owned mask is securely reused and discarded. Uncommon junk jars ought to be set up in networks as brought together removal focuses for the pre-owned masks of occupants. On the off chance that no uncommon trash canisters are accessible, inhabitants could splash disinfectant on the two sides of their pre-owned mask and crease them up before placing them into a fixed plastic pack in the dustbin.

For the security of others and themselves, inhabitants need to deal with their pre-owned mask. Purifying them will help guarantee the pre-owned masks don't turn into a second wellspring of the coronavirus.

Touching Filter Surface

A mask is a worn upside out, just over the nose, not pulled under the jawline, or worn uniquely over the mouth, leaving the nose uncovered. Indeed, even the best mask won't ensure whenever worn mistakenly.

A client was continually contacting and tinkering with the mask's channel surface, which cross-taints fingers and resulting surfaces. A defiled finger will cross-taint the following SEVEN surfaces it contacts, for example, telephones, pads, keypads.

Pulling a face mask under the jaw for discussion or eating, and afterward returning the mask-up once more.

Reusing or reusing masks. This has been a typical and perilous rising practice in Hong Kong since January 2020.

They were wearing a similar mask for a really long time. The period of time that a face mask could be securely worn relies upon the number of individuals a client has been near. The external layer of a mask is a definitive boundary. Like an angling net, it will channel yet additionally gather pathogens, without inactivating or slaughtering them. The more drawn out a mask has been worn around others, the more focused the irresistible burden becomes. A medical mask should not be dressed for more than a day; a specialist or attendant will experience different masks during a solitary work move.

Depending on N95 masks. At the point when worn appropriately, these respirator masks get hot inside and are hard to take in because of the weight change between the air inside and the outside environment. It resembles breathing through a mask and can get upsetting to the client. A client's blood-oxygen immersion can drop and carbon dioxide increments fundamentally with right and delayed use. Indeed, even a sound and fit grown-up could discover wearing an N95, whenever put on effectively, troublesome following an hour or so of utilization. A more seasoned individual or an immunocompromised individual likely would have a hard time utilizing an N95 mask in any event, for a brief timeframe. Wearers may take it off for a break, which would decrease its security. Kids and newborn children are additionally commonly not a suitable possibility for wearing N95s as the danger of suffocation is higher.

CONCLUSION

Protection does not always come easy, but there are some simple ways to keep safe, like making your homemade face masks.

We recommend making 3 masks for everyone: wear one, wash one, and one for storage or sharing. Remember to remove the mask carefully. Do not reach under the mask with dirty hands. Wash your hands and face immediately after removing the mask. For best results cleaning the mask immediately after removing the mask, spray the water with hydrogen peroxide to kill the bacteria, and then wash with soap and warm water.

Best of Luck!